THE ROLE OF MEDICATION IN DIABETES MANAGEMENT

Empowering Patients with Advanced Treatments and Cutting-Edge Solutions"

ANABARAONYE C. FOSTER
MILLICENT NNABUAKU

ISBN-13: 9798327878358
ISBN-10: 1477123456

Cover design by: Art Painter
Library of Congress Control Number: 2018675309
Printed in the United States of America

To all individuals living with diabetes, whose resilience and determination inspire us every day.

To the healthcare professionals, researchers, and caregivers dedicated to advancing diabetes treatment and improving patient lives.

And to our families and friends, for their unwavering support and encouragement on this journey.

This book is for you.

CONTENTS

INTRODUCTION

Diabetes, a chronic metabolic disorder characterized by high levels of blood sugar, has emerged as a global health concern of unprecedented magnitude. With its prevalence steadily rising worldwide, understanding the intricacies of diabetes management becomes increasingly vital. This book, "The Role of Medication in Diabetes Management," endeavors to shed light on the critical nexus between medication and effective diabetes care.

A. Overview of Diabetes:

1. Types of Diabetes:

Diabetes manifests in various forms, each with its unique etiology and management challenges. The primary types include Type 1 diabetes, an autoimmune condition wherein the body's immune system attacks insulin-producing beta cells in the pancreas; Type 2 diabetes, marked by insulin resistance and inadequate insulin production; and Gestational diabetes, a temporary condition that occurs during pregnancy, predisposing both the mother and child to future health risks.

2. Prevalence and Impact:

Diabetes knows no bounds, affecting individuals across age groups, ethnicities, and socio-economic backgrounds. Its prevalence has surged dramatically in recent decades, mirroring trends of sedentary lifestyles, unhealthy dietary habits, and escalating obesity rates. Beyond its sheer prevalence, diabetes exerts a profound impact on health outcomes, contributing significantly to cardiovascular disease, kidney failure, blindness, and lower limb amputations.

B. Importance of Medication in Diabetes Management:

1. Controlling Blood Sugar Levels:

Central to diabetes management is the regulation of blood sugar levels, a delicate balance that hinges on the interplay of diet, exercise, and medication. Medications, ranging from oral drugs to injectable insulin, serve as indispensable tools in this endeavor, facilitating glucose control and mitigating the risk of hyperglycemia-induced complications.

2. Preventing Complications:

Diabetes harbors a litany of potential complications, ranging from neuropathy and nephropathy to cardiovascular disease and retinopathy. By optimizing blood sugar control, medications play a pivotal role in forestalling the onset and progression of these debilitating complications, thereby safeguarding the long-term health and well-being of individuals living with diabetes.

3. Improving Quality of Life:

Beyond its physiological ramifications, diabetes exacts a considerable toll on the psychological and emotional well-being of affected individuals. The burden of managing a chronic condition, coupled with the fear of acute complications, can impede one's quality of life. Herein lies the transformative power of medication, not only in alleviating symptoms and improving metabolic parameters but also in empowering individuals to reclaim agency over their health and lead fulfilling lives.

As we embark on this exploration of the role of medication in diabetes management, we invite readers to delve deeper into the nuances of this multifaceted disease and discover the myriad ways in which medication serves as a cornerstone of effective diabetes care.

CHAPTER I: UNDERSTANDING DIABETES MEDICATION

Effective diabetes management often hinges on the judicious use of medications to regulate blood glucose levels and mitigate the risk of complications. This chapter provides a comprehensive overview of the primary categories of diabetes medications, encompassing both oral and injectable options, and elucidates their mechanisms of action, benefits, and potential side effects.

A. Oral Medications

1. Metformin

Metformin is the cornerstone of Type 2 diabetes treatment. It works primarily by reducing hepatic glucose production and improving insulin sensitivity in peripheral tissues. This dual action helps lower blood glucose levels without causing significant hypoglycemia. Metformin is also known for its favorable impact on weight management and cardiovascular health. Common side effects include gastrointestinal discomfort, which can often be mitigated by gradual dose escalation.

2. Sulfonylureas

Sulfonylureas, such as glipizide and glyburide, function by stimulating the pancreas to produce more insulin. They are effective in lowering blood glucose but carry a higher risk of hypoglycemia and weight gain compared to other oral agents. They are typically used when metformin alone is insufficient to achieve glycemic targets.

3. Thiazolidinediones

Thiazolidinediones (TZDs), including pioglitazone and rosiglitazone, enhance insulin sensitivity in adipose tissue, muscle, and the liver. While effective in improving glycemic control, TZDs are associated with weight gain, fluid retention, and an increased risk of heart failure. Despite these concerns, they remain a viable option for certain patients, particularly those with significant insulin resistance.

4. DPP-4 Inhibitors

Dipeptidyl peptidase-4 (DPP-4) inhibitors, such as sitagliptin and saxagliptin, prolong the action of incretin hormones, which increase insulin release and decrease glucagon secretion in response to meals. DPP-4 inhibitors are generally well-tolerated, with a low risk of hypoglycemia and a neutral effect on weight. However, they may be associated with rare but serious side effects, including pancreatitis.

5. SGLT2 Inhibitors

Sodium-glucose co-transporter-2 (SGLT2) inhibitors, like canagliflozin and empagliflozin, promote the excretion of glucose in the urine by inhibiting its reabsorption in the kidneys. This class of medications not only improves glycemic control but also offers additional benefits such as weight loss and reduced blood pressure. They have been shown to confer cardiovascular and renal protection. Common side effects include genital infections and a risk of diabetic ketoacidosis, particularly in patients with Type 1 diabetes.

B. Injectable Medications

1. Insulin Therapy

Insulin remains a cornerstone for the treatment of Type 1 diabetes and is also essential for many individuals with Type 2 diabetes. There are several types of insulin, categorized by their onset, peak, and duration of action:

I - Rapid-acting insulin (e.g., lispro, aspart): Begins working within minutes and is ideal for mealtime glucose control.

II- Short-acting insulin (e.g., regular insulin): Takes effect within 30 minutes and covers insulin needs for meals eaten within an hour.

III - Intermediate-acting insulin (e.g., NPH): Covers insulin needs for about half a day or overnight.

IV- Long-acting insulin (e.g., glargine, detemir): Provides a steady insulin level to control blood sugar for an entire day.

2 Insulin Delivery Methods:

I- Syringes: Traditional method, requiring manual dose measurement and injection.

II- Pens: Pre-filled or refillable devices offering more convenience and accurate dosing.

III- Pumps: Continuous subcutaneous insulin infusion devices that deliver insulin through a catheter, allowing for precise control and adjustment of insulin delivery.

C. GLP-1 Receptor Agonists

1. Mechanism of Action:

Glucagon-like peptide-1 (GLP-1) receptor agonists, such as exenatide and liraglutide, mimic the action of the incretin hormone GLP-1. They enhance glucose-dependent insulin secretion, suppress glucagon release, slow gastric emptying, and increase satiety.

2. Benefits and Side Effects:

GLP-1 receptor agonists are effective in lowering blood glucose levels and promoting weight loss, making them particularly beneficial for overweight or obese individuals with Type 2 diabetes. They also have a low risk of hypoglycemia when used alone. However, common side effects include gastrointestinal issues such as nausea and vomiting. There are also potential risks of pancreatitis and thyroid tumors, which necessitate careful patient selection and monitoring.

Understanding the diverse landscape of diabetes medications is crucial for tailoring treatment to individual needs and optimizing outcomes. By leveraging the strengths of various oral and injectable therapies, healthcare providers can construct comprehensive management plans that enhance both glycemic control and overall quality of life for people living with diabetes.

CHAPTER II: PERSONALIZING DIABETES MEDICATION REGIMENS

Diabetes management is not a one-size-fits-all endeavor. Individualizing medication regimens is essential to optimize treatment efficacy, minimize side effects, and enhance patient satisfaction. This chapter delves into the critical factors influencing medication choices and underscores the importance of shared decision-making between patients and healthcare providers.

A. Factors Influencing Medication Choices

1. Type of Diabetes

The type of diabetes a patient has significantly impacts the choice of medication. For instance, individuals with Type 1 diabetes require insulin therapy from the onset due to the autoimmune destruction of insulin-producing beta cells. In contrast, those with Type 2 diabetes have a broader spectrum of therapeutic options, including oral medications, non-insulin injectables, and insulin, depending on the severity of insulin resistance and beta-cell dysfunction. Gestational diabetes, occurring during pregnancy, necessitates careful selection of medications that are safe for both the mother and the developing fetus, often prioritizing insulin due to its safety profile.

2. Blood Sugar Levels

The patient's blood glucose levels and HbA1c (glycated hemoglobin) readings are crucial in determining the intensity and type of medication required. For individuals with mild hyperglycemia, lifestyle modifications combined with metformin may suffice. In cases of moderate to severe hyperglycemia, combination therapy with multiple oral agents or the addition of injectable medications may be necessary to achieve target glycemic control.

3. Other Health Conditions

Comorbid conditions play a pivotal role in shaping diabetes treatment plans. For example, patients with heart failure or chronic kidney disease might benefit from SGLT2 inhibitors due to their cardiovascular and renal protective effects. Conversely, thiazolidinediones should be avoided in heart failure patients due to the risk of fluid retention. The presence of other health issues, such as obesity, hypertension, or lipid abnormalities, also guides medication choices to address these concomitant concerns effectively.

4. Lifestyle Factors

A patient's lifestyle, including dietary habits, physical activity levels, and daily routines, influences the selection of diabetes medications. Medications that align with the patient's lifestyle and preferences are more likely to be adhered to. For instance, patients with unpredictable meal schedules might benefit from flexible insulin regimens or GLP-1 receptor agonists that offer mealtime and basal control. Lifestyle factors also encompass psychosocial aspects, such as the patient's ability to manage complex medication regimens and their support systems.

B. Shared Decision Making with

Healthcare Providers

1. Importance of Patient Education

Educating patients about their condition and treatment options is fundamental to effective diabetes management. Understanding the mechanisms, benefits, and potential side effects of prescribed medications empowers patients to make informed decisions. Education also encompasses training on self-monitoring of blood glucose, recognizing symptoms of hyperglycemia and hypoglycemia, and implementing lifestyle modifications to complement pharmacotherapy.

2. Goal Setting and Monitoring

Collaborative goal setting between patients and healthcare providers is vital for personalizing diabetes care. Establishing realistic and achievable targets for blood glucose levels, HbA1c, weight, and other health metrics helps guide treatment decisions and adjustments. Regular monitoring and follow-up appointments allow for the assessment of progress towards these goals, facilitating timely modifications to the medication regimen based on the patient's response and changing needs.

3. Adherence Strategies

Medication adherence is a cornerstone of successful diabetes management. Strategies to enhance adherence include simplifying medication regimens, using fixed-dose combinations to reduce pill burden, and incorporating medications with favorable dosing schedules. Addressing barriers to adherence, such as medication costs, side effects, and patient forgetfulness, through tailored interventions like financial assistance programs, side effect management, and reminder tools (e.g., apps, pillboxes) can significantly improve adherence rates. Encouraging patient engagement and building a supportive healthcare relationship also play critical roles in fostering adherence and long-term management success.

Personalizing diabetes medication regimens requires a nuanced understanding of individual patient factors and a collaborative approach to care. By considering the type of diabetes, blood sugar levels, comorbidities, and lifestyle factors, and by engaging patients through education, goal setting, and adherence strategies, healthcare providers can optimize treatment outcomes and enhance the overall quality of life for individuals living with diabetes.

CHAPTER III: MANAGING MEDICATION SIDE EFFECTS AND COMPLICATIONS

Diabetes medications are essential for maintaining blood glucose control, but they can come with a range of side effects and potential complications. Effective management of these issues is crucial to ensure the safety and well-being of patients. This chapter explores common side effects, strategies to minimize them, and approaches to recognizing and addressing severe complications.

A. Common Side Effects of Diabetes Medications

1. Hypoglycemia:

Hypoglycemia, or low blood sugar, is a frequent side effect of insulin and sulfonylureas. Symptoms include shakiness, sweating, confusion, and, in severe cases, loss of consciousness. It often results from mismatched insulin doses, skipped meals, or excessive physical activity.

2. Weight Gain:

Some diabetes medications, particularly insulin and thiazolidinediones, are associated with weight gain. This can be counterproductive, especially in Type 2 diabetes patients, where weight management is a critical component of treatment.

3. Gastrointestinal Issues:

Gastrointestinal side effects are common with metformin and GLP-1 receptor agonists. These can include nausea, diarrhea, and abdominal discomfort. While often transient, they can affect patient adherence to the medication regimen.

B. Strategies to Minimize Side Effects

1. Lifestyle Modifications

I- Diet: Eating balanced meals at regular intervals can help stabilize blood sugar levels and prevent hypoglycemia. Incorporating high-fiber foods can also alleviate gastrointestinal discomfort.

II- Exercise: Regular physical activity helps manage weight and improve insulin sensitivity. However, exercise routines should be planned to prevent hypoglycemia, especially when using insulin or sulfonylureas.

III- Hydration: Staying well-hydrated can mitigate some gastrointestinal side effects and support overall metabolic function.

2. Medication Adjustments

I- Dosing: Adjusting the timing and dosage of medications can help manage side effects. For example, starting metformin at a low dose and gradually increasing it can reduce gastrointestinal symptoms.

II- Formulations: Switching to extended-release formulations can minimize side effects. Extended-release metformin, for example, is often better tolerated than immediate-release versions.

III- Combination Therapy: Using combination therapies can sometimes reduce the dosage of individual drugs, thereby minimizing side effects. For instance, combining metformin with a DPP-4 inhibitor can improve glycemic control with fewer gastrointestinal issues.

3. Alternative Therapies

I- Herbal Supplements: Some patients explore herbal supplements like cinnamon or berberine for blood sugar control. While not substitutes for prescription medications, they can complement conventional therapy. However, these should be used cautiously and under medical supervision due to potential interactions.

II- Mind-Body Practices: Techniques like yoga and meditation can help reduce stress, which in turn can improve blood sugar control and reduce reliance on higher doses of medication.

C. Recognizing and Addressing Medication Complications

1. Diabetic Ketoacidosis (DKA)

DKA is a serious complication primarily seen in Type 1 diabetes but can occur in Type 2 as well. It results from a severe lack of insulin, leading to high blood sugar and the breakdown of fat for energy, producing ketones. Symptoms include high blood sugar, ketones in urine, rapid breathing, and confusion. Immediate medical intervention is required, often involving fluid replacement, insulin therapy, and electrolyte management.

2. Hyperosmolar Hyperglycemic State (HHS)

HHS is a life-threatening condition more common in Type 2 diabetes, characterized by extremely high blood sugar levels without significant ketosis. Symptoms include severe dehydration, confusion, and lethargy. Treatment focuses on rehydration, insulin administration, and electrolyte balance. Early recognition and intervention are crucial to prevent severe outcomes.

3. Drug Interactions

Many diabetes medications can interact with other drugs, potentially altering their effectiveness or increasing the risk of adverse effects. For example, certain blood pressure medications can mask symptoms of hypoglycemia. Patients should provide a comprehensive list of all medications, including over-the-counter drugs and supplements, to their healthcare providers. Regular review and consultation can help manage and prevent harmful interactions.

Effectively managing the side effects and complications of diabetes medications involves a proactive approach that includes lifestyle modifications, thoughtful medication adjustments, and alternative therapies. Recognizing the signs of serious complications like DKA and HHS and understanding potential drug interactions are critical for maintaining patient safety and achieving optimal therapeutic outcomes. By adopting these strategies, patients and healthcare providers can work together to ensure a balanced and effective diabetes management plan.

CHAPTER IV: INTEGRATING MEDICATION WITH LIFESTYLE MANAGEMENT

Effective diabetes management goes beyond medication. It requires a holistic approach that integrates medication with lifestyle modifications to optimize blood sugar control and overall health. This chapter highlights the importance of diet and exercise, explores complementary therapies, and emphasizes the role of monitoring blood sugar levels in managing diabetes.

A. Importance of Diet and Exercise

1. Dietary Approaches

Proper nutrition is foundational in diabetes management. Several dietary approaches have been shown to benefit individuals with diabetes:

I- Low-Carb Diet: Reducing carbohydrate intake helps lower blood sugar levels. Low-carb diets emphasize protein, healthy fats, and non-starchy vegetables while limiting grains, sugars, and high-carb fruits. This approach can improve glycemic control and assist with weight loss.

II- Mediterranean Diet: This diet focuses on whole grains, lean proteins (especially fish), healthy fats (like olive oil), fruits, and vegetables. It is rich in fiber and antioxidants, which help in managing blood sugar levels and reducing cardiovascular risks associated with diabetes.

III- DASH Diet: The Dietary Approaches to Stop Hypertension (DASH) diet is rich in fruits, vegetables, whole grains, and low-fat dairy, with reduced saturated fat and cholesterol. Originally designed to manage blood pressure, it also helps improve insulin sensitivity and overall metabolic health.

2. Physical Activity Guidelines

Regular physical activity enhances insulin sensitivity, aids in weight management, and improves cardiovascular health. The American Diabetes Association (ADA) recommends:

I- Aerobic Exercise: At least 150 minutes per week of moderate-intensity aerobic activity (e.g., brisk walking, cycling) spread over at least three days, with no more than two consecutive days without exercise.

II- Resistance Training: Engaging in resistance exercises (e.g., weightlifting, resistance bands) at least two to three times per week to build muscle strength and improve glucose uptake.

III- Flexibility and Balance: Activities like stretching, yoga, and tai chi to enhance flexibility, balance, and overall well-being.

B. Complementary Therapies

1. Herbal Supplements

Some herbal supplements have shown potential in supporting diabetes management. Examples include:

I- Cinnamon: May help improve insulin sensitivity and lower blood glucose levels.

II- Berberine: An active compound in several plants, shown to reduce blood sugar and improve lipid metabolism.

III- Fenugreek: Contains soluble fiber that may help lower blood sugar levels.

While promising, herbal supplements should be used with

caution and under healthcare provider supervision due to potential interactions with medications.

2. Mind-Body Practices

I- Yoga: Incorporates physical postures, breathing exercises, and meditation. Yoga can reduce stress, enhance insulin sensitivity, and improve overall metabolic health.

II- Meditation: Regular meditation helps lower stress levels, which can positively impact blood sugar control. Mindfulness-based stress reduction (MBSR) has been particularly effective for individuals with diabetes.

C. Monitoring Blood Sugar Levels

1. Self-Monitoring

Regular self-monitoring of blood glucose (SMBG) is crucial for understanding how various factors like diet, exercise, and medication affect blood sugar levels. SMBG involves using a blood glucose meter to check levels at different times of the day, especially before and after meals, and before bedtime. Keeping a log of these readings helps patients and healthcare providers make informed decisions about treatment adjustments.

2. Continuous Glucose Monitoring (CGM)

Continuous Glucose Monitoring (CGM) systems provide real-time data on blood sugar levels throughout the day and night. CGM devices use a small sensor inserted under the skin to measure glucose levels in interstitial fluid. They offer several advantages:

I- Trend Analysis: CGM provides trend data, showing how blood glucose levels fluctuate over time, which can help identify patterns and triggers of high or low blood sugar.

II- Alerts: Many CGM systems have alarms that notify users of impending hypoglycemia or hyperglycemia, allowing for prompt corrective action.

III- Improved Management: By offering a comprehensive view of glucose trends, CGM helps patients and healthcare providers make more precise adjustments to medication, diet, and activity.

Integrating medication with lifestyle management is vital for effective diabetes care. A balanced diet, regular physical activity, and the inclusion of complementary therapies can significantly enhance medication efficacy and improve overall health outcomes. Consistent monitoring of blood sugar levels, whether through self-monitoring or advanced CGM technology, is essential for maintaining optimal glycemic control and preventing complications. By adopting a holistic approach, individuals with diabetes can achieve better control over their condition and improve their quality of life.

CHAPTER V: OVERCOMING BARRIERS TO MEDICATION ADHERENCE

Adherence to medication regimens is critical for effective diabetes management, yet many patients encounter significant barriers that impede their ability to follow prescribed treatments consistently. Understanding and addressing these barriers is essential to enhance adherence and achieve better health outcomes. This chapter explores common patient perspectives that hinder adherence and outlines strategies to overcome these challenges.

A. Understanding Patient Perspectives

1. Fear of Side Effects

Many patients are apprehensive about potential side effects of diabetes medications. Fear of hypoglycemia, weight gain, gastrointestinal issues, and other adverse effects can lead to intentional non-adherence or reluctance to initiate therapy. Patients may also fear long-term consequences or have had previous negative experiences with medications, influencing their willingness to follow prescribed regimens.

2. Cost Concerns

The financial burden of diabetes medications, including copayments, deductibles, and out-of-pocket expenses, can be prohibitive for many patients. High costs may lead to rationing medication, skipping doses, or forgoing treatment altogether. This is particularly challenging for individuals without adequate health insurance or those facing economic hardships.

3. Complexity of Medication Regimens

Complex medication regimens, involving multiple drugs with different dosing schedules, can be overwhelming and confusing for patients. This complexity increases the risk of missed doses, incorrect administration, and reduced adherence. Patients with busy lifestyles, cognitive impairments, or limited health literacy may find it particularly challenging to manage intricate treatment plans.

B. Strategies for Improving Adherence

1. Simplifying Regimens

I- Combination Pills: Utilizing combination pills that contain multiple medications in a single tablet can reduce the number of pills patients need to take, simplifying their regimen and improving adherence.

II- Fixed Dosing Schedules: Aligning medication dosing schedules with daily routines (e.g., once-daily dosing) can make it easier for patients to remember and adhere to their treatment plans.

III- Medication Management Tools: Tools such as pill organizers, medication reminder apps, and automated dispensers can help patients keep track of their medications and reduce the likelihood of missed doses.

2. Addressing Financial Barriers

I- Generic Alternatives: Prescribing generic versions of medications can significantly reduce costs while providing the same therapeutic benefits as brand-name drugs.

II- Assistance Programs: Informing patients about pharmaceutical assistance programs, discount cards, and local or national resources that help cover medication costs can alleviate financial strain.

III- Insurance Navigation: Assisting patients in understanding their insurance coverage and navigating insurance benefits can help minimize out-of-pocket expenses and identify cost-saving opportunities.

3. Providing Support and Education

I- Patient Education: Educating patients about the importance of medication adherence, potential side effects, and strategies for managing those side effects can empower them to take control of their treatment. Clear communication about the benefits of adherence and addressing misconceptions can also improve compliance.

II- Support Systems: Establishing a support system that includes healthcare providers, family members, and peer support groups can provide emotional and practical support. Regular follow-ups, counseling, and motivational interviewing can help address adherence challenges and encourage patients to stay on track.

III- Tailored Interventions: Customizing interventions to fit individual patient needs and preferences, considering cultural, linguistic, and personal factors, can enhance the effectiveness of adherence strategies. Personalized care plans that align with the patient's lifestyle and values are more likely to be followed consistently.

Improving medication adherence is a multifaceted endeavor that requires understanding and addressing the diverse barriers faced by patients. By simplifying regimens, mitigating financial burdens, and providing robust support and education, healthcare providers can help patients overcome these challenges and achieve better diabetes management. Enhanced adherence not only improves glycemic control but also reduces the risk of complications, ultimately leading to a higher quality of life for individuals with diabetes.

CHAPTER VI: EMERGING TRENDS AND FUTURE DIRECTIONS

The landscape of diabetes management is continuously evolving, driven by advancements in medications, technology, and efforts to address healthcare disparities. This chapter explores the latest developments and future directions that hold promise for improving the care and outcomes for individuals with diabetes.

A. Advancements in Diabetes Medications

1. Novel Drug Classes

Recent years have seen the development of several novel drug classes that offer new mechanisms of action and potential benefits for diabetes management:

I- GLP-1/GIP Receptor Agonists: These dual agonists, such as tirzepatide, target both GLP-1 and glucose-dependent insulinotropic polypeptide (GIP) receptors, providing enhanced glycemic control and significant weight loss compared to existing therapies.

II- Immunomodulatory Drugs: For Type 1 diabetes, research is focusing on drugs that modulate the immune system to preserve or restore pancreatic beta-cell function. Examples include teplizumab, which targets specific immune cells to delay the onset of Type 1 diabetes in high-risk individuals.

III- SGLT1/2 Inhibitors: Combining SGLT1 and SGLT2 inhibition, these drugs enhance glucose excretion through the kidneys and also delay glucose absorption in the intestines, offering dual benefits for blood sugar control and weight management.

2. Personalized Medicine Approaches

Personalized medicine aims to tailor treatment based on individual genetic, metabolic, and phenotypic characteristics:

I- Pharmacogenomics: Understanding genetic variations that affect drug metabolism and response can guide the selection of the most effective and safest medications for each patient.

II- Biomarkers: Identifying biomarkers that predict treatment response or risk of complications enables more precise and personalized treatment plans, potentially improving outcomes and reducing adverse effects.

B. Technology and Diabetes Management

1. Artificial Pancreas Systems

The artificial pancreas, also known as an automated insulin delivery system, combines continuous glucose monitoring (CGM) with an insulin pump, using sophisticated algorithms to automate insulin delivery:

I- Improved Glycemic Control: These systems continuously adjust insulin doses based on real-time glucose readings, maintaining blood sugar levels within the target range more effectively than manual methods.

II- Enhanced Quality of Life: By reducing the burden of constant blood sugar monitoring and insulin adjustments, artificial pancreas systems improve the quality of life for individuals with diabetes.

2. Closed-Loop Insulin Delivery

Closed-loop systems represent an advanced form of artificial pancreas technology:

I- Dual-Hormone Systems: These systems administer both

insulin and glucagon, mimicking the pancreas's natural regulatory mechanisms to prevent both hyperglycemia and hypoglycemia.

II- Adaptive Algorithms: Continuous learning algorithms that adapt to individual patterns of glucose fluctuations and insulin sensitivity improve the accuracy and efficacy of insulin delivery over time.

C. Addressing Healthcare Disparities

1. Access to Medications

Ensuring equitable access to diabetes medications is crucial for effective management across diverse populations:

I- Affordable Medications: Efforts to reduce the cost of diabetes medications through generic alternatives, price negotiations, and patient assistance programs are essential to prevent cost-related non-adherence.

II- Distribution Networks: Expanding distribution networks to reach underserved areas, including rural and low-income urban communities, ensures that all patients have access to necessary medications and supplies.

2. Cultural and Socioeconomic Factors

Addressing cultural and socioeconomic disparities involves tailored strategies to meet the unique needs of diverse populations:

I- Culturally Competent Care: Training healthcare providers in cultural competence ensures that they can effectively communicate with and understand the needs of patients from different cultural backgrounds. This includes respecting dietary preferences, language barriers, and cultural beliefs about health and illness.

II- Community-Based Interventions: Engaging community health workers and local organizations to provide education, support, and resources can improve diabetes management in socioeconomically disadvantaged groups. Programs that address social determinants of health, such as food security, housing stability, and access to healthcare, are critical for comprehensive diabetes care.

The future of diabetes management is bright, with ongoing advancements in medications and technology promising to improve outcomes and quality of life for individuals with diabetes. Addressing healthcare disparities ensures that these innovations benefit all patients, regardless of their socioeconomic status or cultural background. By embracing these emerging trends and future directions, the healthcare community can make significant strides toward better diabetes care and a healthier future for those affected by this chronic condition.

CHAPTER VII: CONCLUSION

A. **Recap of Key Points**

The management of diabetes is multifaceted, requiring a careful balance of medication, lifestyle modifications, and continuous monitoring. This book has explored the critical role that medication plays in controlling blood sugar levels, preventing complications, and improving the quality of life for individuals with diabetes. We have delved into the various types of diabetes and their distinct management needs, highlighting the importance of personalizing medication regimens to suit individual patient profiles. Understanding diabetes medications, including oral and injectable options, is essential for tailoring treatments effectively. Addressing medication side effects and integrating lifestyle management are key to achieving comprehensive diabetes care. Additionally, overcoming barriers to medication adherence and keeping abreast of emerging trends and future directions in diabetes management are vital for ongoing success in this field.

B. **Empowering Patients in Diabetes Management**

Empowering patients is central to effective diabetes management. Education plays a crucial role in helping patients understand their condition and the medications they are prescribed. By fostering open communication between patients and healthcare providers, we can ensure that treatment plans are both effective and manageable. Shared decision-making encourages patients to take an active role in their care, leading to better adherence and outcomes. Providing support, whether through patient education, financial assistance programs, or simplified medication regimens, helps patients overcome obstacles and manage their diabetes more effectively. Empowered patients are more likely to make informed choices, adhere to their treatment plans, and adopt healthy lifestyle changes that complement their medication regimens.

C. Looking Towards the Future of Diabetes Care

The future of diabetes care is promising, with ongoing advancements in medications and technology set to revolutionize management strategies. Novel drug classes and personalized medicine approaches are paving the way for more targeted and effective treatments. Technological innovations, such as artificial pancreas systems and closed-loop insulin delivery, offer the potential for more precise and automated blood sugar control. Addressing healthcare disparities remains a critical focus, ensuring that all individuals, regardless of socioeconomic or cultural background, have access to the latest advancements in diabetes care.

As we look towards the future, continued research and development will be crucial in uncovering new therapies and improving existing ones. Integrating these innovations into everyday practice will require collaboration between healthcare providers, researchers, policymakers, and patients. By staying informed and adaptable, we can navigate the evolving landscape of diabetes management and work towards a future where optimal care and improved outcomes are accessible to all.

In conclusion, the role of medication in diabetes management is indispensable. Combined with lifestyle modifications, patient education, and cutting-edge technology, medications form the cornerstone of effective diabetes care. Empowering patients and addressing healthcare disparities will ensure that these advancements benefit everyone, leading to a brighter future for individuals living with diabetes.

ACKNOWLEDGEMENT

We extend our heartfelt gratitude to everyone who contributed to the creation of this book, "The Role of Medication in Diabetes Management."

First and foremost, we thank the patients and their families, whose courage and perseverance inspire our work. Your stories and experiences have shaped our understanding of diabetes management and motivated us to strive for better care.

To our colleagues in the medical and research communities, your collaborative spirit and dedication to advancing diabetes treatment have been invaluable. We are especially grateful to the healthcare professionals who generously shared their insights and expertise, enriching the content of this book.

We also wish to acknowledge the support of our respective institutions and organizations, which have provided the resources and encouragement necessary to bring this project to fruition. Your commitment to improving healthcare outcomes for those living with diabetes is deeply appreciated.

A special thank you to our editorial team and publishers, whose guidance and meticulous attention to detail have been instrumental in refining this manuscript. Your professionalism and dedication have ensured that our message is clear and impactful.

To our families and friends, your unwavering support and patience have been our anchor throughout this journey. Your belief in our mission has been a constant source of strength and motivation.

Finally, we dedicate this book to the ongoing quest for better diabetes management and to all those who continue to work tirelessly to improve the lives of individuals with diabetes. Together, we can make a difference.

With deepest gratitude,

Anabaraonye C. Foster and Millicent Nnabuaku

ABOUT THE AUTHOR

Anabaraonye C. Foster   Millicent Nnabuaku

Anabaraonye C. Foster

Anabaraonye C. Foster is a renowned diabetes educator and healthcare advocate with over two decades of experience in the field. With a background in clinical pharmacology and a passion for patient education, Foster has dedicated his career to improving the lives of those living with diabetes. His expertise in medication management and his commitment to personalized patient care have earned him recognition in both medical and patient communities. Foster is also a sought-after speaker at international conferences and a prolific writer, contributing to numerous medical journals and publications. His practical insights and compassionate approach make him a trusted voice in diabetes management.

Millicent Nnabuaku

Millicent Nnabuaku is a distinguished endocrinologist and researcher, specializing in diabetes and metabolic disorders. With a deep commitment to advancing diabetes care, Nnabuaku has conducted groundbreaking research on innovative treatment approaches and the impact of lifestyle modifications on diabetes management. Her work has been published in prestigious medical journals, and she frequently collaborates with global health organizations to improve diabetes care standards worldwide. Nnabuaku is also a dedicated mentor and educator, empowering patients and healthcare professionals with knowledge and tools to effectively manage diabetes. Her holistic approach and dedication to addressing healthcare disparities make her a leading advocate for equitable diabetes care.

Together, Foster and Nnabuaku bring a wealth of knowledge and experience to "The Role of Medication in Diabetes Management," offering readers practical advice, cutting-edge insights, and a compassionate understanding of the challenges and triumphs in diabetes care.